The 6-Week Endo-Diet Plan That Changed My Life

By

Susan J. Derek

The 6-Week Endo-Diet Plan That Changed My Life

Copyright © 2023 by Susan J. Derek

Before this book is not to be duplicated or reproduced in any manner without the publisher's consent. Therefore, the content is not to be stored electronically, transferred, or kept in a database. The content is not to be kept in parts and is not to be copied, scanned, faxed or retained without the approval of the publisher or creator.

TABLE OF CONTENTS

PART 1 6

INTRODUCTION 6

CHAPTER 1 8

UNDERSTANDING ENDOMETRIOSIS
....8

1.1 What Is Endometriosis? 8

1.2 The Impact of Endometriosis on Women's Lives 8

1.3 The Need for a Specialized Diet 9

PART II 11

PREPARING FOR THE 11

ENDO-DIET 11

CHAPTER 2 12

UNDERSTANDING NUTRITION BASICS 12

2.1 The Role of Nutrition in Managing Endometriosis 12

2.2 Key Nutrients for Endo-Sufferers.....13

2.3 Recognizing Trigger Foods 14

PART III 16

THE DIET PLAN 16

CHAPTER 3 17

UNDERSTANDING ENDO-DIET 17

Why Does the Endo-Diet Matter? 17

Key Principles of the Endo-Diet: 17

CREATING YOUR MEAL PLAN 18

PART IV 20

CHAPTER 4 22

ANTI-INFLAMMATORY FOODS........22

CHAPTER 5 34

HORMONES-RELATED FOODS 34

Hormones and Endometriosis..................34

Hormones Involved in Endometriosis: ...34

Foods for Hormone Balance 35

Flaxseed and Berry Smoothie...................35
Kale and Chickpea Salad..........................36
Baked Salmon with Turmeric Quinoa.....36
Greek Yogurt with Berries and Almonds
....37
CHAPTER 6..39
GUT HEALTH AND HEALING............39
The Gut Microbiome: 39
Inflammation and Gut Health:................39
Foods for Gut Health 40
Greek Yogurt Parfait 41
Quinoa and Chickpea Salad.....................41
Homemade Kimchi 42
PART IV 43
MONITORING 43
AND ADAPTING 43
CHAPTER 7..44
KEEPING A FOOD JOURNAL 44

Advantages of Maintaining a Food Journal **45**

PART IV **46**

SUCCESS STORIES AND INSPIRATIONAL INTERVIEWS **46**

CHAPTER 8 ....**47**

REAL-LIFE ENDO-DIET **47**

SUCCESS STORIES............................**47**

Story 2: Mike's Journey to Supporting His Partner..**49**

Story 3: Ava's Journey to Self-Discovery **49**

CONCLUSION **52**

PART 1
INTRODUCTION

An agonizing pain that I had never before felt gripped my abdomen. I recall that day very clearly because it was the start of a new chapter in my life when I learned that I had endometriosis.

I experienced various emotions as the doctor described the illness. Anxiety, and rage overcame me. It hit me like a ton of bricks that I would be fighting this chronic illness. I had no idea how much it would alter my life.

In the years that followed, there were many medical check-ups, operations, and prescription drugs. Endometriosis had a vice-like grip on my life, causing both physical pain and wreaking havoc on my psychological well-being. I felt caught in a ceaseless pattern of torment, uneasiness, and depression.

However, there was a glimmer of hope in the gloom. My doctor acquainted me with a specialized diet and exercise plan custom-fitted to oversee endometriosis side effects. It was a beam of daylight getting through the tempestuous mists, promising help and an opportunity for a superior life.

In the pages of this book, I will share with you the very plan that transformed my life—the 6-Week Endo-Diet. This comprehensive program that was carefully developed by medical professionals gave me a lifeline when I most needed it. I started to experience notable changes within six weeks, including decreased pain, increased energy, and an improved sense of body control.

I invite you to join me on this journey, whether you're dealing with the difficulties of endometriosis or just want to learn more about this condition. As you read this book and follow the meal plan, I can assure you that significant changes will occur. Armed with knowledge, perseverance, and the power of exercise and nutrition, we will work together to navigate the world of endometriosis.

Welcome to the 6-Week Endo-Diet Plan—a journey of hope, healing, and transformation.

CHAPTER 1

UNDERSTANDING ENDOMETRIOSIS

In the world of women's health, there exists a quiet, frequently misconstrued lowlife known as endometriosis. This chapter is committed to disentangling the secrets encompassing this condition, a condition that influences a huge number of ladies all over the planet and that turned into a defining chapter in my own life story.

1.1 What Is Endometriosis?

Endometriosis is a chronic, frequently painful medical condition that develops when endometrium, tissue that normally lines the uterus, starts to grow outside of the uterus. While a more definite clarification of what endometriosis is can be tracked down in my book *"Healing*

Journey: How I Overcame Endometriosis in 6 Weeks," it's essential to grasp the fundamentals here as well.

1.2 The Impact of Endometriosis on Women's Lives

Endometriosis can cause brutal symptoms. It doesn't stop there; for many, it means enduring agonizing pelvic pain, especially during menstruation. Other distressing symptoms can result from the condition, such as:

Constant pelvic agony*:* A constant, pulsating hurt that can influence day-to-day existence.

Torment during intercourse: a feeling that is extremely unsettling and can strain relationships.

Weighty feminine dying: frequently accompanied by crippling cramps.

Problems with the gut: such as gas, constipation, and diarrhea.

Fatigue: Depleting energy levels and influencing everyday exercises.

Infertility: a devastating outcome for some.

In any case, in addition to the actual side effects, endometriosis is so challenging. The profound cost is similarly critical. Numerous ladies with endometriosis experience dissatisfaction, uneasiness, sadness, and a feeling of confinement. The unending suffering and uncertainty of the future can have a serious negative impact on mental health.

1.3 The Need for a Specialized Diet

I started to realize how crucial nutrition is to managing endometriosis as I struggled with my own diagnosis. It wasn't just about managing symptoms; It had to do with taking back control of my life. I discovered that while some foods can numb and help my body heal, others can make inflammation and pain worse. The foundation of my recovery journey was this knowledge.

In the accompanying chapters, we will explore in detail the dietary changes and meal plans that became my lifeline, changing my life from one of agony and despondency to one of hope and vitality.

PART II
PREPARING FOR THE ENDO-DIET

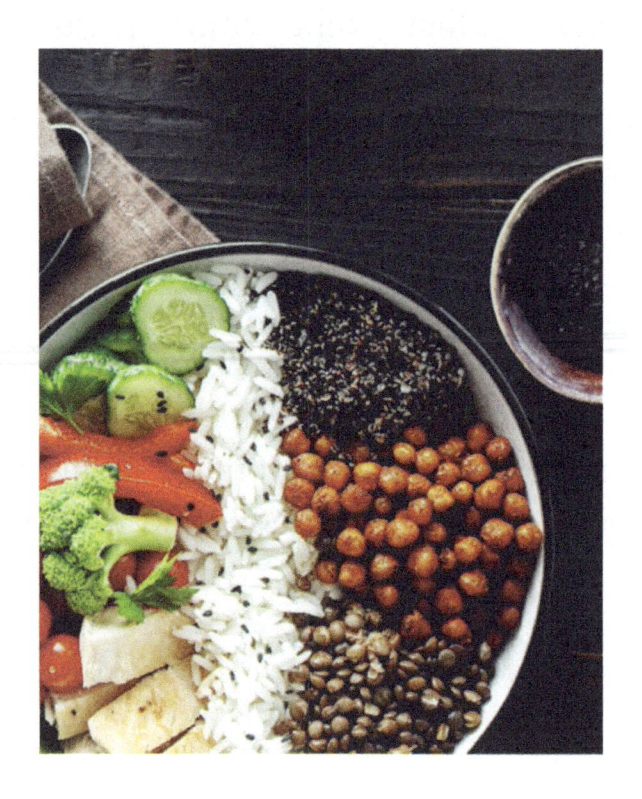

CHAPTER 2

UNDERSTANDING NUTRITION BASICS

In our journey to overcome endometriosis and recapture control of our wellbeing, understanding the basics of nourishment is a vital initial step. This section is devoted to divulging the science behind sustenance and its significant effect on endometriosis symptoms. You will be able to make well-informed choices on your way to wellness with this knowledge.

2.1 The Role of Nutrition in Managing Endometriosis

Nutrition isn't just about satisfying hunger; it's an incredible asset for managing endometriosis. The food sources we devour can either fuel our side effects or lessen them. Let's investigate the impact of nutrition on endometriosis.

Chronic inflammation: Endometriosis is frequently associated with chronic inflammation, which produces pain and other symptoms. Certain foods can either speed up or slow down inflammation. We'll identify which foods fall into each category.

Hormone Balance: Hormones have a big impact on endometriosis. Nutrition can have an impact on hormonal changes. Recognize the foods that support hormone balance.

Nutrient Deficiencies: Endo-sufferers frequently lack particular nutrients. Discover the fundamental nutrients and minerals that can assist with tending to these inadequacies.

2.2 Key Nutrients for Endo-Sufferers

Endometriosis sufferers have been found to benefit especially from certain nutrients. We will investigate these nutrients, their roles in the management of symptoms, and the foods that supply them:

Fatty Acids Omega-3: These beneficial fats are effective anti-inflammatory agents. Discover how to incorporate omega-3s into your diet and the best sources.

Fiber: Fiber supports digestion and regulate hormones. Find out about high-fiber food sources that can ease gastrointestinal side effects.

Antioxidants: Antioxidants reduce inflammation and combat oxidative stress. Learn about the numerous antioxidant-rich foods and how to incorporate them into your daily diet.

2.3 Recognizing Trigger Foods

Similarly, as specific food sources can help those with endometriosis, others can be impeding, intensifying side effects and aggravation. It's fundamental to perceive these trigger food sources and comprehend the reason why they ought to be restricted or stayed away from.

Some endo-sufferers say that cutting back on gluten helped. We'll investigate the connection among gluten and endometriosis side effects.

Dairy: For some people, dairy products can cause inflammation. We'll talk about the advantages of dairy alternatives.

Foods Processed: Exceptionally handled food sources frequently contain added substances that can compound side effects.

Figure out how to detect and stay away from these secret guilty parties.

As we embark on the 6-Week Endo-Diet plan, this comprehension of nutrition basics will act as the establishment for your journey to better wellbeing. You will be better able to make dietary choices that support your well-being and alleviate symptoms armed with this information. Keep in mind that nutrition is more than just what you eat; It's about having the ability to change your life and get rid of endometriosis, one meal at a time.

PART III
THE DIET PLAN

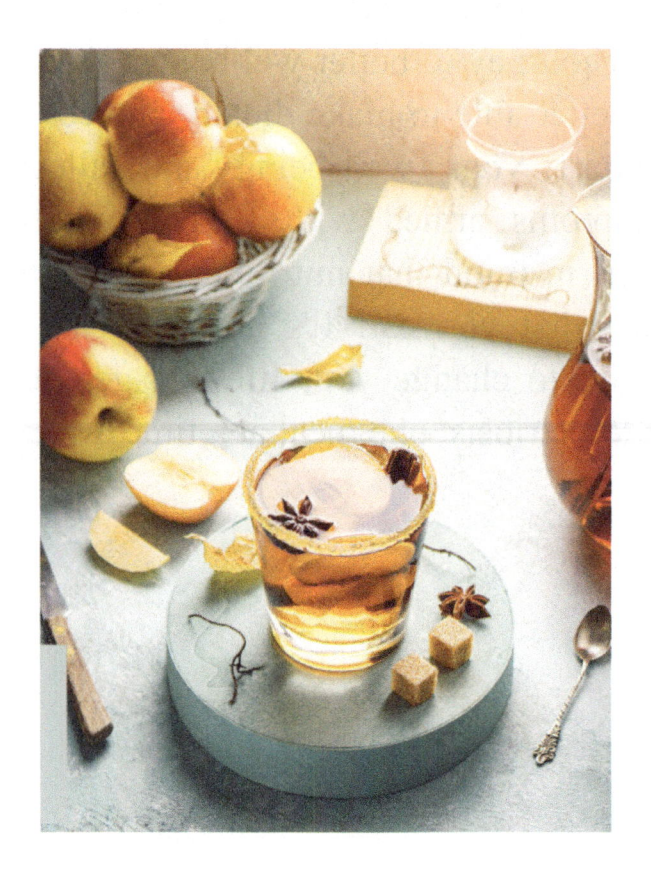

CHAPTER 3
UNDERSTANDING ENDO-DIET

The Endo-Diet is a specialized eating plan that promotes a balanced and anti-inflammatory diet to alleviate endometriosis symptoms. It centers around food varieties that can assist with lessening irritation, control hormones, and backing generally well-being. This diet is not a one-size-fits-all plan; rather, it is a framework that you can modify to meet your specific requirements and preferences.

As you progress further in this book, you will discover recipes I adopted that resulted to a 6-week significant positive changes in my entire health.

Why Does the Endo-Diet Matter?

The growth of tissue outside the uterus that is similar to the uterine lining is a characteristic of endometriosis. It can cause extreme torment, weighty periods, and fertility issues. The goal of the Endo-Diet is to get rid of inflammation and hormonal imbalances, two major causes of endometriosis symptoms. By making mindful food choices, you can potentially find relief and improve your quality of life.

Key Principles of the Endo-Diet:

Balanced nutrition: The Endo-Diet emphasizes balanced meals that incorporate an assortment of nutrition types to provide essential nutrients.

Anti-Inflammatory Foods: Numerous endometriosis side effects are connected to irritation. Anti-inflammatory foods are the main focus of the diet.

Hormone Regulation: Menstrual pain and mood swings can be reduced by eating certain foods that help regulate hormone levels.

Whole Foods: Processed and sugary foods are minimized, while whole, unprocessed foods take center stage.

Careful Eating: Eating mindfully and paying attention to portion sizes can help control symptoms and manage weight.

CREATING YOUR MEAL PLAN

Now that you have an understanding of the Endo-Diet's core principles, it's time to understand some factors to consider when creating your meal plan.

Step 1: Assess Your Current Diet

Take stock of your eating habits right away. What foods do you typically consume daily? Are there any foods that cause or exacerbate your symptoms like the foods mentioned under trigger foods?

If you know where you started, it will be easier to make specific changes.

Step 2: Identify Endo-Diet Foods

Learn about the foods that are recommended for the Endo-Diet by becoming familiar with them. These include:

Vegetables, whole grains (like brown rice, quinoa, and oats), lean proteins (like chicken, fish, and tofu), healthy fats (like avocado, olive oil, and nuts), dairy alternatives (like almond milk and coconut yogurt), and herbs and spices (like ginger and turmeric)

Step 3: Plan Your Meals

Based on your assessments, plan your meals around foods that impedes the effect of endometriosis.

The 6-Week Endo-Diet Plan That Changed My Life

The 6-Week Endo-Diet Plan That Changed My Life

PART IV
THE RECIPES

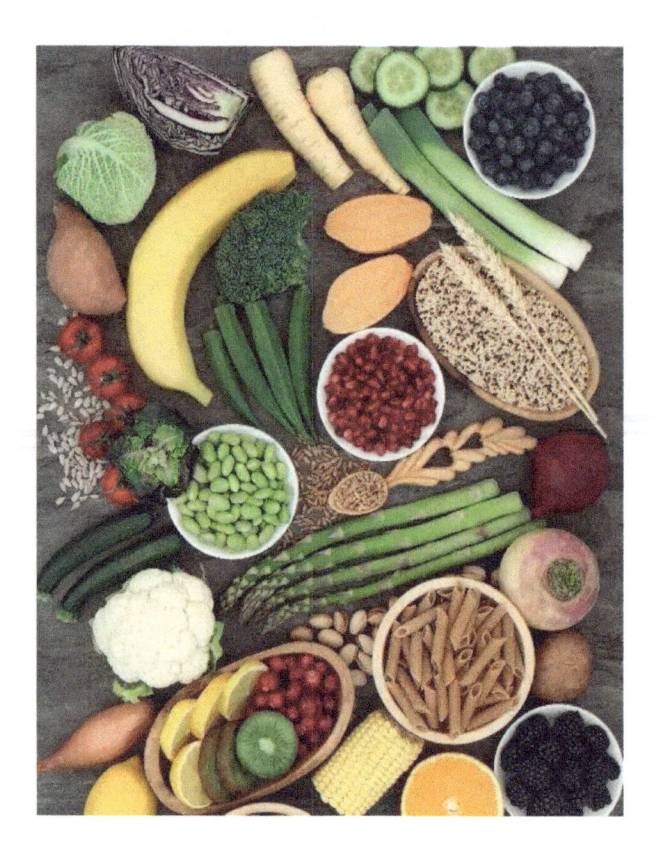

CHAPTER 4
ANTI-INFLAMMATORY FOODS

Anti-inflammatory foods were part of my plan during the 6-week diet plan following insights garnered from professional medical experts as the anti-inflammatory properties help in reducing to a large extent my pains and inflammation associated with the condition.

Here are some:

1. Nutrient-Packed Smoothie Bowl:

The smoothie bowl contains turmeric, which is known for its calming properties. Curcumin, a potent anti-inflammatory ingredient, can be found in turmeric.

Ingredients:

- 1 cup of unsweetened almond milk
- 1/2 cup of frozen berries (such as blueberries or strawberries)

- 1/2 ripe banana
- 1 tablespoon of chia seeds
- 1 tablespoon of flax seeds
- 1 teaspoon of turmeric powder
- 1 teaspoon of honey (optional)

Guidelines:

- Blend all the ingredients until smooth.

Turmeric is known for its anti-inflammatory properties, which can help reduce the pain associated with endometriosis.

2. Ginger-Turmeric Tea:

Ingredients:
1-inch piece of fresh ginger, sliced
1 teaspoon of ground turmeric
2 cups of water
Honey or lemon for flavor (optional)

Guidelines:

- Bring water to a boil and add ginger and turmeric.
- Simmer for 10-15 minutes.
- Strain the tea into a cup and add honey or lemon if desired.

Ginger and turmeric both have anti-inflammatory properties and may help reduce pain and inflammation.

3. Salmon and Quinoa Bowl:

Ingredients:
4 oz of grilled salmon
1 cup of cooked quinoa
1 cup of steamed broccoli
1/2 avocado, sliced
Drizzle with lemon juice.

Guidelines:

- Place the cooked quinoa in a bowl.
- Arrange avocado slices, steamed broccoli, and grilled salmon on top.
- Apply fresh lemon juice to the dish.

Salmon is rich in omega-3 unsaturated fats, which have anti-inflammatory properties. Quinoa is rich in nutrients and fiber.

4. Spaghetti Squash with Pesto:

Spaghetti squash is an alternative to pasta that is low in carbs and contains vitamins and fiber. Pesto, which is made from basil and olive oil, adds flavor, healthy fats, contains compounds that have anti-inflammatory properties. This dish is easy to prepare and can be a nutritious option for those with endometriosis.

Ingredients:

For the Spaghetti Squash:

- 1 medium-sized of spaghetti squash
- Olive oil
  Salt and pepper to taste

For the Pesto Sauce:

- 2 cups of fresh basil leaves
- 1/2 cup of grated Parmesan cheese (or nutritional yeast for a dairy-free option)
- 1/2 cup of pine nuts or walnuts (toasted)
- 2-3 cloves of garlic
- 1/2 cup of extra virgin olive oil
- Salt and pepper to taste

- Lemon juice (optional, for added flavor)

Guidelines:

For the Spaghetti Squash:

- Set the oven temperature to 375°F (190°C).
- Cut the spaghetti squash in half lengthwise after washing it.
- Using a spoon, remove the pulp and seeds from the center.
- Brush the cut sides of the squash with olive oil and sprinkle with salt and pepper.
- Place the squash parts, cut side down, on a baking sheet lined with parchment paper.
- Broil the squash in the preheated stove for around 35-45 minutes, or until the flesh is tender and easily

shreds into spaghetti-like strands when scraped with a fork. Cooking time may vary depending upon the size of the squash.
- Let the cooked squash cool slightly after taking it out of the oven.
- Scrape the flesh with a fork after it has cooled to make strands that look like spaghetti. Place the strands in a different bowl.

For the Pesto Sauce:

- In a food processor, consolidate the basil leaves, grated Parmesan cheese (or dietary yeast), toasted pine nuts or pecans, and garlic cloves.
- The ingredients should be pulsed until they are finely chopped.
- While the food processor is running, gradually drizzle in the extra virgin

olive oil until the mixture comes together into a smooth paste.
- Salt, pepper, and a squeeze of lemon juice can be added to taste to the pesto. Adjust the seasonings to your preference.

Assembly:

Mix the pesto sauce with the cooked spaghetti squash strands. Use as much or as little pesto as you prefer.

Serve the Spaghetti Squash with Pesto warm, decorated with extra grated Parmesan cheese or nutritional yeast, whenever wanted.

This dish isn't just delightful yet additionally rich in anti-inflammatory ingredients like basil, olive oil, and garlic. It is a great option for endometriosis sufferers and can be adapted to suit individual taste preferences. Enjoy!

5. Roasted Vegetable Stir-Fry:

A variety of nutrients and fiber can be found in a stir-fry made with roasted vegetables. You can utilize *tofu or tempeh* as a plant-based protein source. The stir-fry sauce's ginger and garlic may have anti-inflammatory properties, which may help alleviate pain caused by endometriosis.

Ingredients:

For the Roasted Vegetables:

- 2 cups of mixed vegetables (e.g., bell peppers, broccoli, carrots, snow peas, and zucchini)
- 2 tablespoons of olive oil
- Salt and pepper to taste
- 1 teaspoon of minced garlic
- For the Stir-Fry Sauce:

- 2 tablespoons of low-sodium soy sauce or tamari (for a gluten-free choice)
- 1 tablespoon of honey or maple syrup (adjust to taste)
- 1 teaspoon of grated ginger
- 1 teaspoon of cornstarch or arrowroot powder (to thicken the sauce)
- 1-2 tablespoons of water (as needed for the desired consistency)

For the Stir-Fry:

- 1 cup of protein of choice (e.g., tofu, tempeh, or cooked chicken or shrimp if preferred)
- Cooked brown rice, quinoa, or rice noodles (optional, for serving)

Guidelines:

For the Roasted Vegetables:

- Preheat your oven to 425°F (220°C).
- Wash, peel (if necessary), and cut the mixed vegetables into bite-sized pieces.
- Toss the vegetables with olive oil, minced garlic, salt, and pepper in a large mixing bowl until well coated.
- On a parchment-lined baking sheet, evenly distribute the vegetables.
- Roast the vegetables in the preheated oven for about 20–25 minutes, or until they are delicate and marginally caramelized, blending partially through for cooking.
- After the vegetables have been roasted, remove them from the oven and set them aside.

For the Stir-Fry Sauce:

Grate ginger, low-sodium soy sauce or tamari, honey or maple syrup, and cornstarch or arrowroot powder are all combined in a small bowl until well combined. Assuming the sauce is excessively thick, you can add 1-2 tablespoons of water to reach the ideal consistency.

For the Stir-Fry:

- Olive oil can be added to a large skillet or wok over medium-high heat.
- Add the protein (tofu, tempeh, cooked chicken or shrimp) to the skillet and cook until it is heated through and lightly browned. Set the protein aside after removing it from the skillet.
- In the same skillet, add the roasted vegetables.

- Pour the stir-fry sauce over the vegetables and toss to coat. he sautéed food sauce over the vegetables and throw to cover. Cook an additional two to three minutes, or until the vegetables are coated in the sauce and it thickens,
- In the event that you removed the protein earlier, add it back to the skillet and mix to consolidate.
- Serve the Roasted Vegetable Stir-Fry over cooked brown rice, quinoa, or rice noodles if desired.

The roasted vegetables in this dish provide a lot of fiber, vitamins, and minerals, and the stir-fry sauce is delicious. It can be made with the protein of your choice and served with whole grain or rice substitute. Endometriosis sufferers can enjoy a well-balanced and nutritious meal thanks to this adaptable recipe.

6. Avocado-Grilled Chicken Salad:

This salad is a protein-rich feast that incorporates barbecued chicken and solid fats from avocado. Monounsaturated fats, which can help reduce inflammation, can be found in abundance in avocado. The salad also incorporates fresh vegetables for added nutrients and fiber.

Ingredients:

For the Barbecued or Grilled Chicken:

- 2 boneless, skinless chicken bosoms
- 2 tablespoons of olive oil
- Salt and pepper to taste
- 1 teaspoon of dried Italian flavoring (optional)

For the Salad:

- Salad greens, such as lettuce, spinach, and arugula
- one ripe avocado, sliced
- Cherry tomatoes, halved
- Cucumber sliced
- Thinly sliced red onion
- Any other desired salad vegetables, such as bell peppers and carrots.

For the Dressing:

- 3 tablespoons of additional virgin olive oil
- 2 tablespoons of balsamic vinegar
- 1 teaspoon of Dijon mustard
- 1 clove of garlic, minced
- Salt and pepper to taste

Guidelines:

For the Grilled Chicken:

- Use a grill pan on the stove or heat your grill to medium-high temperature.
- Combine the olive oil, salt, pepper, and dried Italian seasoning (if using) in a small bowl.
- Make sure the chicken breasts are well-coated by brushing them with the olive oil mixture.
- Put the chicken bosoms on the preheated barbecue or barbecue dish and cook for around 6-8 minutes for every side, or until they are cooked through with no pink in the middle. Depending on the thickness of the chicken breasts, the cooking time may vary.
- After the chicken has finished cooking, take it off the grill and let it rest for a few minutes. After that, slice it into bite-sized or thin strips.

For the Salad:

Mix the mixed salad greens, sliced avocado, cherry tomatoes, cucumber, red onion, and any other desired salad vegetables together in a large salad bowl.

For the Dressing:

Combine the extra virgin olive oil, balsamic vinegar, Dijon mustard, minced garlic, salt, and pepper in a small bowl with a whisk until well combined.

Assembly:

- Toss the dressing over the salad and toss gently to coat the vegetables.
- Layer the grilled chicken slices on top of the salad.

- As an immediate meal, serve your Grilled Chicken Salad with Avocado with crusty bread or whole-grain rolls if you prefer.

Fresh vegetables, healthy fats from the avocado, and lean protein from the grilled chicken make this salad a healthy and balanced option for people with endometriosis. The homemade dressing adds flavor without requiring excessive amounts of unhealthy fats or added sugar. Take pleasure in your nutritious meal!

CHAPTER 5
HORMONES-RELATED FOODS

Before we delve into the main theme of this chapter, it is of immense importance we understand the relationship between hormones and endometriosis.

Hormones and Endometriosis

Endometriosis is a complicated condition impacted by hormonal imbalances in the body. The menstrual cycle is regulated by hormones like estrogen, and when these hormones are out of balance, endometrial tissue outside the uterus can grow and multiply, resulting in pain and other endometriosis symptoms.

Understanding the interplay of hormones in endometriosis is essential for managing the condition effectively. While the Endo-Diet can't fix endometriosis completely, it can help rebalance hormones, possibly decreasing side effects and working on your overall quality of life.

Hormones Involved in Endometriosis:
1. Estrogen:

Estrogen is primarily responsible for the growth and thickening of the endometrial lining in preparation for menstruation.

In endometriosis, there can be an abundance of estrogen or an irregularity among estrogen and progesterone, prompting tissue excess.

2. Progesterone:

The second half of the menstrual cycle is controlled by progesterone.

Endometrial tissue growth may be aided by an imbalance in estrogen and progesterone.

3. Insulin:

Endometriosis symptoms can be made worse by elevated insulin levels, which can trigger an increase in estrogen production.

Managing glucose levels is essential for chemical equilibrium.

Foods for Hormone Balance

Diet can be a powerful tool for balancing hormones in endometriosis management. Consider these important dietary practices during my season of tackling endometriosis.

Flaxseed and Berry Smoothie

Ingredients:

- 1 cup unsweetened almond milk
- 1 tablespoon ground flaxseeds

- 1/2 cup blueberries, strawberries, and raspberries
- 1/2 banana
- 1 teaspoon honey (optional)

Guidelines:

Blend all ingredients until smooth, and enjoy a nutritious and hormone-balancing breakfast.

Kale and Chickpea Salad

Ingredients:

- 2 cups chopped kale leaves
- 1 cup cooked chickpeas
- 1/4 cup diced red bell pepper
- 1/4 cup shredded carrots
- 2 tablespoons olive oil and lemon juice dressing
- Salt and pepper to taste

Guidelines:

Mix all of the ingredients together for a lunch that balances hormones and tastes good.

Baked Salmon with Turmeric Quinoa
Ingredients:

- 2 salmon filets
- 1 teaspoon turmeric powder
- 1 cup quinoa
- 2 cups vegetable broth
- 1 cup broccoli florets
- Lemon wedges for embellish

Guidelines:

- Season salmon with turmeric, salt, and pepper. Bake for about 15-20 minutes at 375°F (190°C).
- In a different pot, cook quinoa in vegetable stock.

- Steam broccoli until tender.
- Steamed broccoli and salmon should be served with turmeric quinoa on top. Garnish with lemon wedges.

Greek Yogurt with Berries and Almonds
Ingredients:

- 1/2 cup Greek yogurt
- 1/4 cup blended berries
- 1 tablespoon cut almonds

Guidelines:

Top Greek yogurt with berries and almonds for a satisfying and hormone-balancing nibble.

Other hormone related foods you can consider are fiber-rich foods like whole grains, legumes, and plenty of fruits and vegetables. Also, herbal teas like chasteberry (vitex) and spearmint. You may also consider lean protein sources like poultry, tofu, and legumes, etc

Being regularly hydrated helps flush toxins from your body and supports overall hormonal health.

CHAPTER 6
GUT HEALTH AND HEALING

There is a connection between your gut and endometriosis and this must be taken seriously. The management of endometriosis symptoms and overall health are significantly influenced by gut health. There's a strong connection between the gut and endometriosis, and understanding this link can help you make informed dietary choices.

The Gut Microbiome:

The gut microbiome alludes to the trillions of microscopic organisms and different microorganisms dwelling in your gastrointestinal system. Digestive processes, nutrient absorption, and immune system regulation all depend on these microorganisms. An imbalance in the gut microbiome, known as dysbiosis, can add to aggravation and compound endometriosis symptoms.

Inflammation and Gut Health:

Endometriosis is related with chronic irritation, and the stomach is a central part in the body's provocative reaction. Inflammation throughout the body can be exacerbated by a ill-fitting gut, which may exacerbate endometriosis symptoms. Thusly, supporting a sound stomach is fundamental for dealing with the condition.

Foods for Gut Health

In my 6-week Endo-Diet plan, I focused on food varieties and dietary practices that help a sound stomach. Here are key procedures to advance stomach or gut wellbeing:

1. Foods High in Fiber:

Fiber upholds the development of helpful stomach microbes. Eat a diet rich in fruits, vegetables, legumes, and whole grains.

2. Foods High in Probiotics:

Beneficial bacteria that support gut health are known as probiotics. Incorporate aged food varieties like yogurt, kefir, sauerkraut, and kimchi in your meals.

3. Prebiotic foods:

Fibers in food called prebiotics help the good bacteria in your gut thrive. Food varieties like garlic, onions, leeks, asparagus, and bananas are rich in prebiotics.

4. Bone Broth:

Bone broth contains amino acids and collagen that can assist with recuperating the stomach lining and diminish irritation.

5. Foods that reduce inflammation: Food sources wealthy in cancer prevention agents, like berries, mixed greens, and turmeric, assist with diminishing stomach aggravation.

Let's consider some recipes under the above categories that help in strengthening gut health.

Greek Yogurt Parfait
Ingredients:

- 1 cup of Greek yogurt
- 1/2 cup of blended berries
- 1 tablespoon full of honey
- 2 tablespoons full of granola

Guidelines:

In a glass, layer granola, honey, mixed berries, and Greek yogurt.

Quinoa and Chickpea Salad
Ingredients:

- 1 cup cooked quinoa
- 1/2 cup cooked chickpeas
- 1/4 cup diced cucumber
- 1/4 cup cherry tomatoes, divided
- 2 tablespoons olive oil and lemon juice dressing
- New spices (mint or parsley) for garnish

Guidelines:

For a mouthwatering and satiating meal, combine all ingredients and garnish with fresh herbs.

Homemade Kimchi
Ingredients:

1 small Napa cabbage, chopped

2 tablespoons Korean red pepper flakes (gochugaru)

2 cloves garlic, minced

1-inch piece of ginger, grated

1 tablespoon fish sauce (optional for umami)

Guidelines:

Mix all ingredients in a bowl, ensuring the cabbage is coated with the spice mixture.

Pack the mixture into a glass jar, pressing it down to remove air bubbles.

Seal the jar and leave it at room temperature for 1-2 days to ferment. Refrigerate after fermentation.

PART V
MONITORING AND ADAPTING

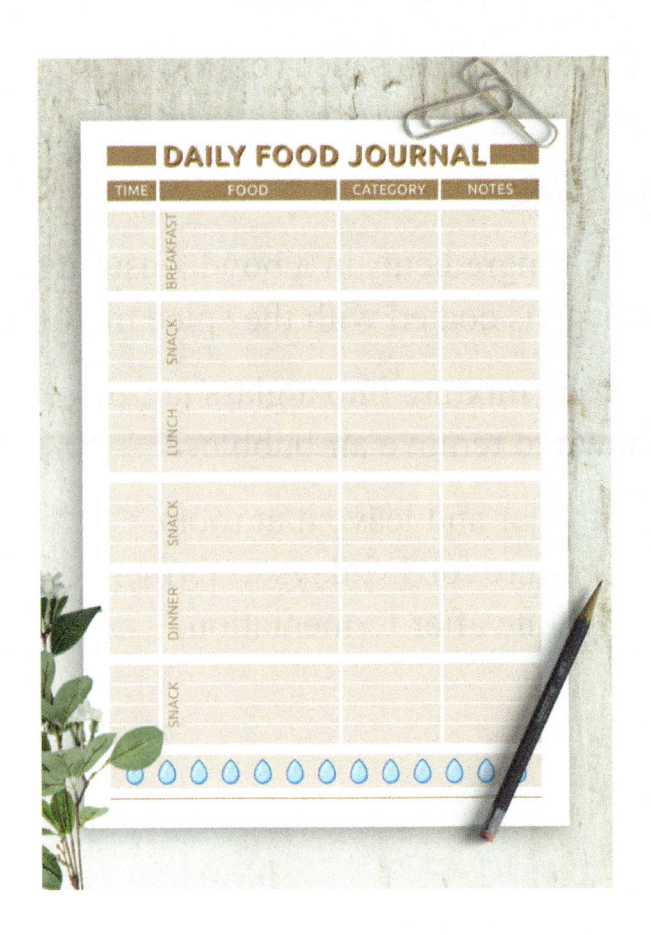

CHAPTER 7
KEEPING A FOOD JOURNAL

During my journey with the Endo-Diet, keeping a food journal was a powerful tool. It permitted me to track my meals, symptoms, and overall well-being, providing valuable insights into how my diet affects my endometriosis. These are factors I thought about while making one.

Select a Journal Design: You can utilize an actual journal, a cell phone application, or a computerized calculation sheet to record your food consumption.

Write everything down: Keep track of everything you consume throughout the day, including the ingredients and portion sizes.

Include Monitoring of Symptoms: In addition to your meals, note any endometriosis symptoms you experience each day. Be specific about the kind of pain, fatigue, bloating, or other symptoms, as well as how bad they are.

Timing is crucial: Be sure to record how long you eat each meal and snack. This may assist in identifying correlations between your symptoms and diet.

Note: In case you need the exact journal template I adopted, you can check it out on amazon with the keyword *'My Endo-Diet Journal'*.

Advantages of Maintaining a Food Journal

Identify Triggers: As patterns develop over time, it may become clear which particular foods or behaviors are causing or exacerbating your symptoms.

Track Progress: By keeping an eye on your symptoms, you can determine whether your condition is getting better or whether dietary changes are having a positive effect.

Work with Medical Professionals: If you choose to speak with a doctor, your food journal can be a helpful tool you can share with them to help with diagnosis and treatment.

PART VI
SUCCESS STORIES AND INSPIRATIONAL INTERVIEWS

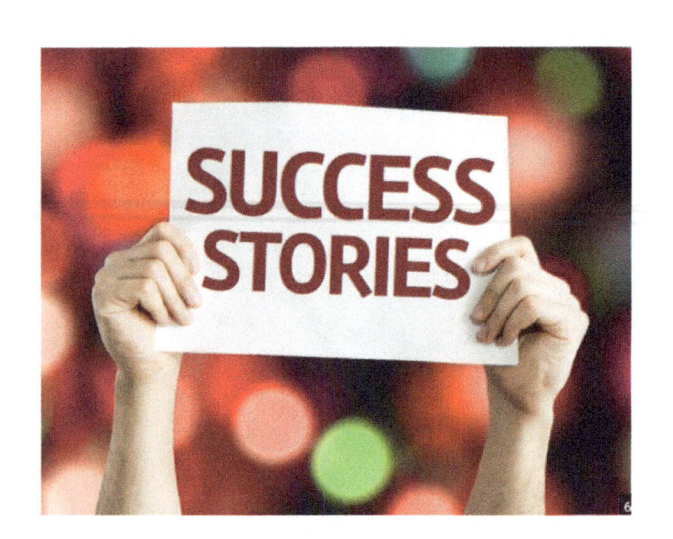

CHAPTER 8
REAL-LIFE ENDO-DIET SUCCESS STORIES

For nearly five years, I have successfully conquered endometriosis, and during this time, I have shared my personal journey with those facing the same challenge. I have guided them through the path that led to my recovery, which aligns with the content I've shared in this book and in my previous work titled ***'Healing Journey: How I Overcame Endometriosis in Six Weeks.'*** The stories of success resulting from my guidance have been numerous, and I will share some of these inspiring tales in this chapter.

If you are interested in obtaining a copy of 'Healing Journey: How I Overcame Endometriosis in Six Weeks,' you can find it available for purchase on Amazon.

Story 1: Tonia's Quest for Better Health

Meet Tonia, a 32-year-old who, like many others, dealt with the difficulties of having endometriosis every day. Due to her severe pain, frequent periods, and extreme weariness, Tonia looked for alternatives to traditional medical care.

Tonia looked into alternate methods of controlling her endometriosis because she was determined to enhance her quality of life. She read about my experience with the Endo-Diet and was motivated by it. Tonia made the decision to adopt the Endo-Diet and adhere to the recommendations I provided in my book, "Healing Journey: How I Overcame Endometriosis in six Weeks," after seeing the potential advantages.

Tonia's life started to improve as she religiously adhered to the Endo-Diet recommendations and made wise eating decisions. She started eating nutrient-dense meals, placed a high priority on gut health, and worked toward hormonal balance. Even though she faced obstacles along the way, she stayed dedicated to the procedure.

Tonia's general wellbeing seen notable improvements over time. Her energy levels increased, and her discomfort and bloating improved. Her endometriosis symptoms were reduced as a result of this good change, which also gave her more energy and self-confidence.

Tonia's experience is evidence of the Endo-Diet's capacity to enhance endometriosis sufferers' lives and effect positive change. Her experience serves as a reminder of the value of tenacity, dedication, and a supportive dietary strategy in treating this illness.

Story 2: Mike's Journey to Supporting His Partner

Endometriosis has an influence on loved ones of individuals who have it as well as those who have it themselves. Mike, an understanding husband, saw Emily deal with the difficulties of endometriosis on a daily basis. He learned about the Endo-Diet in one of my free online seminars and was determined to assist Emily in any way he could.

Together, Mike and Emily started their nutritional adventure by taking nutrition classes and preparing balanced meals as learnt in my seminar. They stopped eating manufactured food and concentrated on utilizing organic, complete foodstuffs. Emily started to feel better, and the pain and discomfort subsided.

Their relationship was reinforced by Mike's steadfast support and dedication to the Endo-Diet, and together they embraced a healthier lifestyle. Emily's development not only raised her standard of living but also deepened the bond between her and Mike.

Story 3: Ava's Journey to Self-Discovery

I originally met Ava through a close friend of hers when I was looking for a distinctive piece of artwork to decorate my office. I had no idea that our first connection would develop into a transforming journey for Ava, guided by my own experience.

Ava, a gifted artist who was 27 years old, was not only a soul full of creativity but also a fighter fighting endometriosis. Her enthusiasm for painting had suffered as a result of her daily battles with pain, weariness, and irritability. She appeared to have lost the spark that formerly drove her creativity as a result of her illness.

During one of our conversations about art and life, Ava learned of my own triumph over endometriosis through the Endo-Diet. She was inspired by my narrative and anxious to investigate the possibilities it presented. Ava made the decision to embark on a journey of self-discovery in the hopes of reviving her creative spirit.

I started collaborating with Ava to modify the Endo-Diet to fit her lifestyle. She adopted a new dietary regimen that placed an emphasis on nutrient-dense foods, promoted intestinal health, and sought to balance hormones. I served as her mentor and advisor, imparting my wisdom and experiences while providing direction and support at every turn.

Over time, the effects of Ava's dietary transformation became evident not only in her physical well-being but also in her creative resurgence. Her suffering and discomfort subsided, and she rediscovered her love of painting. Her health had significantly improved thanks to the Endo-Diet, and her artistic expression had undergone a tremendous metamorphosis.

Ava is now a free woman, no longer constrained by the restrictions endometriosis formerly placed on her life.

CONCLUSION

As we come to an end with "The 6-Week Endo-Diet Plan That Changed My Life," let me take this opportunity to extend my sincere compliments for your commitment to bettering your health and wellbeing. Together, we've looked at a revolutionary nutritional strategy that might improve your overall quality of life and help you manage the symptoms of endometriosis.

We've gone into the complexities of the Endo-Diet throughout this book, discussing things like balanced nutrition, gut health, hormone balance, and self-discovery. You now possess a plethora of information and useful skills that will help you proceed through your trip with assurance and fortitude.

It's important to recognize that the journey you've undertaken is not merely a temporary fix or a short-term solution.

Instead, the Endo-Diet and the meal plans offered here are intended to fit seamlessly into your lifestyle and promote your long-term wellbeing.

Though the Endo-Diet and meal plans are intended to be a permanent part of your life, it's important to keep in mind that noticeable benefits are frequently seen within the first 6 weeks. This period of time acts as a potent introduction to the potential advantages of this dietary strategy, giving an idea of what is possible with commitment and mindful eating.

Remember that every little change you've made matters when you look back on your path. Your dedication to controlling endometriosis and enhancing your health is evidence of your fortitude and adaptability. Though your early weeks may have seen the most visible outcomes, your ongoing transformation is a lifelong journey full of opportunities.

I appreciate you joining me on this transforming path. May you thrive, explore, and change as you go, knowing that you have the ability to create a better and healthier future for yourself.

Made in the USA
Las Vegas, NV
24 September 2024